**Lose 10kg in 2 Months
Never Feel Hungry Dieting**

By Nkiru Ojimadu

This is an

Ojimadu Books Publications

I dedicate this book to my mum - Queen Anastasia
"Arukaakwa" Ojimadu. Continue to rest in the Lord,
Mummy!

P.S. Please read till the end to understand the changes in you as they happen.

Contents

Introduction

Disclaimer : I am not a dietician or a medical doctor. In this book I will share with you actions that I took that made me and many that I coach through the years lose tons of weight and still keep them.

So I suggest that before you start executing any of the plans I shared here please consult your doctor.

That said, my name is Nkiru Ojimadu, friends and family fondly call me Niki. I am a life transformational coach. One of my main passions is for men and women live to their full potential. It is actually much more difficult to do this if you are overweight.

As the book title suggests, I had a journey to get to where I am today physically and in general as well.

When I just got married, my weight was 60 kilograms with the height of 1.72metres with 90-60-90 shape until the children started coming.
I have 3 children after my 1st, 2nd and 3rd babies, my shape and weight went back to normal. However, 5 years after my last child, I had a stillbirth. It was horrible. I believe my stomach never went back to normal and due to abrupt removal of the dead fetus, my hormonal imbalance was out of control due to this I gained a lot of weight. I gained 30 kilograms!

I never paid any attention to the weight gain at that time because I was in a community of girls, who due to their culture believed that as a married woman with 3 children, I was in perfect shape. I felt so good and bought their complements for a long time until I left that community.

It was after I joined another community of ladies that were generally slim and believed that, having three children is not a license to weight gain. That was when I really noticed how big I was. Don't ever underestimate the power and the influence of your environment.

Please don't misunderstand me if you are big, like I was. However, whether you are big or slim, you must love yourself the way you are but that does not mean that you should not work on yourself and strive to be better. Love yourself the way you are but become a better you. Strive to be better .

One other thing that motivated me to write this book is, the last days of my mum on earth. Mummy was big and this caused a lot of health issues along the line. Issues like high blood pressure, diabetes and so on. Can slim people have similar issues like my mum? Yes, they can, but the difference is, if you are slim, you make very much easier for those that take care of you to handle your weight. It was not easy for mummy and for everyone that was taking care of her. Continue to rest in peace dearest mummy.

So my dear reader, do your best to eat healthy and be in shape. This is one of the ways you show love to yourself, your friends and family.

Strive to be better, strive to be healthier. How you can achieve that and more are exactly what you will learn from this book.

If you take your time to study and practice all that is written here, you will be amazed by your results. You would not only lose 10 kg but, will lose as much as you desire by giving yourself more time. People have used this plan to lose up to 50 kg in 6 months and more.

Now let's dig in!

Our Guts Are Our 2nd Brains.

The secret of losing weight comes from your digestive health

In general these five sets of food help a great deal in shedding off those fats and keeping your stomach flat.

1. Food containing high probiotics.(Healthy, live microorganisms - mainly bacteria and yeasts - that contribute to the health of the gut, the metabolism of nutrients, and the flow of the digestive system. Probiotics build a microbiome, and are found in gastrointestinal tracts and certain foods, including yogurt. Recently, supplements containing probiotics are a new source of these beneficial microorganisms.)

2. Food high in fiber

3. Food high in water

4. Food containing high prebiotics (Prebiotics are defined as "nondigestible food ingredients that beneficially affect the host by selectively stimulating the growth of one or a limited number of bacterial species in the colon, such as Bifidobacteria and Lactobacilli, which have the potential to improve host health." Prebiotics are, simply speaking, the "food" for beneficial bacteria.)

5. Certain herbs and spices

What we put in there will determine how all the other parts of the body works. You are what you eat and how you eat it.

- Rushing your food

- Skipping meals

are two main factors that help NOT to lose weight.

These three questions will help you eliminate some foods from your diet:

- Do I feel weak, tired and bloated as soon as I finish eating?
- Do I always feel lack of energy?
- Do I always struggle with losing weight despite cutting down on calories and regular exercise?

These questions will help you determine which food to eat which not to.

What Type Of Weight Loss Program Is Sensible?

Weight loss programs need to be :
- Easy
- Effective
- Enjoyable

Before you start, ask yourself these questions
- Do I have any illnesses: Hormonal, liver, kidney, issues, climax, gynecological problems?
- Did I have any surgical operations?
- How much weight do I want to lose?

- When do I want to lose the weight?. (Give yourself a realistic time frame). For example: if you tell yourself , "Hey , I need to lose 20 kilograms of my bodyweight in three days" . Well, you might get your goal met but is not a healthy way to lose weight and most probably you will gain back 40kg!

If you have any health issues consult your doctor to know which of the advice given below you should avoid. However if all is normal, if you have no health issues , let's get started!

Your Plate And Cup.
- Drink four cups of water with lemon, first thing in the morning
- But before lemon with water, I also take a cup of kefir/sour milk with a spoon of ground flaxseed. If you are new in this introduce the flaxseed gradually. Start with a teaspoon. Take a month break from time to time.
- Eat only 45 minutes after that.
- Eat at a time, only the quantity of food that can enter the palms of your hands. That is the size of your stomach.
- Get a small flat plate and use it. It helps to eat small portions at a time.

- However, you should eat a large quantity of vegetables especially green leafy vegetables daily.
- Eat a high-protein breakfast.
- Avoid sugary drinks and fruit juice.
- Drink water a half hour before meals.
- Choose weight loss-friendly foods. I will give a list of weight loss-friendly foods below.
- Eat soluble fiber.
- Beetroot is a must in your daily diet because of it's antioxidant quality.
- Eat mostly whole, unprocessed foods.
- Eat your food slowly
- Chew carrots thoroughly before you go to bed. This helps to scrub your colon while you sleep. I have found this very effective in weight loss

There are many ways to lose a lot of weight fast.

However, most of them will make you hungry and unsatisfied.

If you don't have iron willpower, then hunger will cause you to give up on these plans quickly.

The plan outlined here will:

 Reduce your appetite significantly.
Make you lose weight quickly, without hunger.
Improve your metabolic health at the same time.
Here is a simple 3-step plan to lose weight fast.

1. Cut Back on Sugars and Starches

The most important part is to cut back on sugars and starches (carbs).

These are the foods that stimulate secretion of insulin the most. If you didn't know already, insulin is the main fat storage hormone in the body.

When insulin goes down, fat has an easier time getting out of the fat stores and the body starts burning fats instead of carbs.

Another benefit of lowering insulin is that your kidneys shed excess sodium and water out of your body, which reduces bloat and unnecessary water weight .

It is not uncommon to lose up to 4.5 kilograms / 10 pounds (sometimes more) in the first week of eating this way, both body fat and water weight.

Cut the carbs, lower your insulin and you will start to eat less calories automatically and without hunger.

Put simply, lowering your insulin puts fat loss on "autopilot "

Summary: Removing sugars and starches (carbs) from your diet will lower your insulin levels, kill your appetite and make you lose weight without hunger.

Low-carb dieting versus portion control or calorie counting

Reducing the amount of carbohydrates in your diet is one of the best ways to lose weight.

It tends to reduce your appetite and cause "automatic" weight loss, without the need for calorie counting or portion control.

This means that you can eat until fullness, feel satisfied and still lose weight.

Why Would You Want to do Low-Carb?

For the past few decades, the health authorities have recommended that we eat a calorie restricted, low-fat diet.

The problem is that this diet doesn't really work. Even when people manage to stick to it, they don't see very good results.

An alternative that has been available for a long time is the low-carb diet. This diet restricts your intake of carbohydrates like sugars and starches (breads, pasta, etc.) and replaces them with protein and fat.

Studies show that low-carb diets reduce your appetite and make you eat fewer calories and lose weight pretty much effortlessly, as long as you manage to keep the carbs down.

In studies where low-carb and low-fat diets are compared, the researchers need to actively restrict calories in the low-fat groups to make the results comparable, but the low-carb groups still usually win.

Low-carb diets also have benefits that go way beyond just weight loss. They lower blood sugar, blood pressure and triglycerides. They raise HDL (the good) and improve the pattern of LDL (the bad) cholesterol.

Low-carb diets cause more weight loss and improve health much more than the calorie restricted, low-fat diet still recommended by the mainstream. This is pretty much a scientific fact at this point.

Summary: There are many studies showing that low-carb diets are more effective and healthier than the low-fat diet that is still recommended all around the world.

How to Figure Out Your Need For Carbohydrates

There is no clear definition of exactly what constitutes a "low carb diet" and what is "low" for one person may not be "low" for the next.

An individual's optimal carb intake depends on age, gender, body composition, activity levels, personal preference, food culture and current metabolic health.

People who are physically active and have more muscle mass can tolerate a lot more carbs than people who are sedentary. This particularly applies for those who do a lot of high intensity, anaerobic work like lifting weights or sprinting.

Metabolic health is also a very important factor. When people get the metabolic syndrome, become obese or get type II diabetes, the rules change.

People who fall into this category can't tolerate the same amount of carbs as those who are healthy. Some scientists even refer to these problems as "carbohydrate intolerance."

Summary : The optimal carb range varies between individuals, depending on activity levels, current metabolic health and a bunch of other factors.

Guidelines That Work 90% of The Time

If you simply remove the unhealthiest carb sources from your diet, refined wheat and added sugars, then you'll be well on your way to improved health.

However, to enjoy the full metabolic benefits of low-carbohydrate diets, you also need to restrict other carb sources.

Even though there is no scientific paper that explains exactly how to match carbohydrate intake to individual needs, I have personally found these guidelines to be very effective.

100-150 Grams Per Day

This is more of a "moderate" carbohydrate intake. It is very appropriate for people who are lean, active and simply trying to stay healthy and maintain their weight.

It is very possible to lose weight at this (and any) carb intake, but it may require you to count calories and/or control portions.

Carbs you can eat:

All the vegetables you can imagine.
Several pieces of fruit per day.
Some amount (not a lot) of healthy starches like potatoes, sweet potatoes and healthier grains like rice and oats.

50-100 Grams Per Day

This range is great if you want to lose weight effortlessly while allowing for a bit of carbs in the diet. It is also a great maintenance range for people who are carb sensitive.

Carbs you can eat:

Plenty of vegetables.
Maybe 2-3 pieces of fruit per day.
Minimal amounts of starchy carbohydrates.

20-50 Grams Per Day

This is where the metabolic benefits really start to kick in. This is the perfect range for people who need to lose weight fast, or are metabolically deranged and have obesity or diabetes.

When eating less than 50 grams per day, your body will get into ketosis, supplying energy for the brain via so-called ketone bodies. This is likely to kill your appetite and cause you to lose weight automatically.

Carbs you can eat:

Plenty of low-carb vegetables.
Some berries, maybe with whipped cream (yummy).
Trace carbs from other foods like avocados, nuts and seeds.

Be aware that a low-carb diet is NOT no-carb. There is room for plenty of low-carb vegetables. Personally I had never eaten as many veggies as when I first started on a low-carb diet.

We are all unique and what works for one person may not for the next. It is important to do some self-experimentation and figure out what works for you.

If you have a medical condition then make sure to talk to your doctor before making any changes, because this diet can drastically reduce your need for medication!

Summary: For people who are physically active or want to maintain their weight, a range of 100-150 grams per day may be optimal. For people who have metabolic problems, going under 50 grams per day is a good idea.

Good Carbs, Bad Carbs

A low-carb diet isn't just about weight loss, it is also supposed to improve your health.

For this reason, it should be based on real, unprocessed foods and healthy carb sources.

So-called "low carb junk foods" are a bad choice.

If you want to improve your health, then choose unprocessed foods: meats, fish, eggs, vegetables, nuts, healthy fats and full-fat dairy products.

Choose carbohydrate sources that include fiber. If you prefer a "moderate" carb intake then try to choose unrefined starch sources like potatoes, sweet potatoes, oats, rice and other non-gluten grains. Personally, I prefer mainly buckwheat.

Added sugar and refined wheat are always bad options and should be eliminated or limited.

Summary: It is very important to choose healthy, fiber-rich carb sources. There is room for plenty of vegetables, even at the lowest end of the carb range.

You Will Become a Fat Burning Machine.

Low-carb diets greatly reduce your blood levels of insulin, a hormone that brings the glucose (from the carbs) into cells.

One of the functions of insulin is to store fat. Many experts believe that the reason low-carb diets work so well, is that they reduce your levels of this hormone.

Another thing that insulin does is to tell the kidneys to hoard sodium. This is the reason high-carb diets can cause excess water retention.

When you cut carbs, you reduce insulin and your kidneys start shedding excess water.

It is common for people to lose a lot of water weight in the first few days on a low-carb diet, up to 2,5- 5 kilograms

Weight loss will slow down after the first week, but this time the fat will be coming from your fat stores.

Studies show that low-carb diets are particularly effective at reducing the fat in your abdominal cavity (belly fat), which is the most dangerous fat of all and highly associated with many diseases.

If you're new to low-carb eating, you will probably need to go through an adaptation phase where your body is getting used to burning fat instead of carbs.

This is called the "low-carb flu" and is usually over within a few days. After this initial phase is over, many people report having more energy than before, with no "afternoon dips" in energy that are common on high-carb diets.

Adding more fat and sodium to your diet can help with this.

Summary: It is common to feel suboptimal in the first few days of lowering your carb intake. However, most people feel excellent after this initial adaptation phase.

Take This Home:

1.   Eat Low Carb

One of the great benefits of low-carb diets is that they're ridiculously simple. You don't need to track anything if you don't want to.

Just eat some protein, healthy fats and veggies at every meal. Throw in some nuts, seeds and full-fat dairy products for good measure. Choose unprocessed foods. It doesn't get much simpler than that!

2. Eat Protein, Fat and Vegetables

Each one of your meals should include a protein source, a fat source and low-carb vegetables. Constructing your meals in this way will automatically bring your carb intake into the recommended range of 20-50 grams per day.

Protein Sources:

Meat – Beef, chicken, pork, lamb, bacon, etc.
Fish and Seafood – Salmon, trout, shrimps, lobsters, etc.
Eggs – Omega-3 enriched or pastured eggs are best.
The importance of eating plenty of protein can not be overstated.

This has been shown to boost metabolism by 80 to 100 calories per day.

High protein diets can also reduce obsessive thoughts about food by 60%, reduce desire for late-night snacking by half, and make you so full that you automatically eat 441 fewer calories per day... just by adding protein to your diet.

When it comes to losing weight, protein is the king of nutrients.

Low-Carb Vegetables:

Broccoli
Cauliflower
Spinach
Kale
Brussels Sprouts
Cabbage
Swiss Chard
Lettuce
Cucumber
Celery
etc.

Don't be afraid to load your plate with these low-carb vegetables. You can eat massive amounts of them without going over 20-50 net carbs per day.

A diet based on meat and vegetables contains all the fiber, vitamins and minerals you need to be healthy. There is no physiological need for grains in the diet.

Fat Sources:

Olive oil
Coconut oil
Avocado oil
Butter
Tallow

Eat 2-3 meals per day. If you find yourself hungry in the afternoon, add a 4th meal.

Don't be afraid of eating fat, trying to do both low-carb AND low-fat at the same time is a recipe for failure. It will make you feel miserable and abandon the plan.

The best cooking fat to use is coconut oil. It is rich in fats called Medium Chain Triglycerides (MCTs). These fats are more fulfilling than others and can boost metabolism slightly .

There is no reason to fear these natural fats, new studies show that saturated fat doesn't raise your heart disease risk at all.

In summary: Assemble each meal out of a protein source, a fat source and a low-carb vegetable. This will put you into the 20-50 gram carb range and drastically lower your insulin levels.

3. Lift Weights 3 Times Per Week

You don't need to exercise to lose weight on this plan, but it is recommended.

The best option is to go to the gym 3-4 times a week. Do a warm up, lift weights, then stretch.

If you're new to the gym, ask a trainer for some advice.

By lifting weights, you will burn a few calories and prevent your metabolism from slowing down, which is a common side effect of losing weight .

Studies on low-carb diets show that you can even gain a bit of muscle while losing significant amounts of body fat .

If lifting weights is not an option for you, then doing some easier cardio workouts like running, jogging, swimming or walking will suffice.

In summary : It is best to do some sort of resistance training like weight lifting. If that is not an option, cardio workouts work too.

Optional – Do a "Carb Re-feed" Once Per Week.

You can take one day "off" per week where you eat more carbs. Many people prefer Saturday.

It is important to try to stick to healthier carb sources like oats, rice, quinoa, potatoes, sweet potatoes, fruits, etc.

But only this one higher carb day, if you start doing it more often than once per week then you're not going to see much success on this plan.

If you must have a cheat meal and eat something unhealthy, then do it on this day.

Be aware that cheat meals or carb refeeds are NOT necessary, but they can up-regulate some fat burning hormones like leptin and thyroid hormones.

You will gain some weight during your re-feed day, but most of it will be water weight and you will lose it again in the next 1-2 days.

Summary : Having one day of the week where you eat more carbs is perfectly acceptable, although NOT necessary.

What About Calories and Portion Control?

It is NOT necessary to count calories as long as you keep the carbs very low and stick to protein, fat and low-carb vegetables.

However, if you really want to, then use this calculator.

Enter your details, then pick the number from either the "Lose Weight" or the "Lose Weight Fast" section – depending on how fast you want to lose.

There are many great free tools you can use to track the amount of calories you are eating. Tools like: Cron-o-meter, Fat Secret, MyFitnessPal etc.

The main goal is to keep carbs under 20-50 grams per day and get the rest of your calories from protein and fat.

Summary : It is not necessary to count calories to lose weight on this plan. It is most important to strictly keep your carbs in the 20-50 gram range.

10 Weight Loss Tips to Make Things Easier (and Faster)

Here are 10 more tips to lose weight even faster:

Eat a high-protein breakfast. Eating a high-protein breakfast has been shown to reduce cravings and calorie intake throughout the day.

Avoid sugary drinks and fruit juice. These are the most fattening things you can put into your body, and avoiding them can help you lose weight.

Drink water a 45 minutes to half hour before meals. One study showed that drinking water at least half hour before meals increased weight loss by 44% over 3 months.

Choose weight loss-friendly foods.

Certain foods are very useful for losing fat. Here is a list of the 20 most weight loss-friendly foods on earth.

Eat soluble fiber. Studies show that soluble fibers may reduce fat, especially in the belly area. Fiber supplements like glucomannan can also help.

Drink coffee or tea. If you're a coffee or a tea drinker, then drink not more than three cups daily, ONLY BLACK coffee. Caffeine in them can boost your metabolism by 3-11% . However, there is a downside to this soi I'll rather keep away from coffee.

Eat mostly whole, unprocessed foods. Base most of your diet on whole foods. They are healthier, more filling and much less likely to cause overeating.

Eat your food slowly. Fast eaters gain more weight over time. Eating slowly makes you feel fuller and boosts weight-reducing hormones.

Use smaller plates. Studies show that people automatically eat less when they use smaller plates. Strange, but it works. Eat lots of vegetables though.

Get a good night's sleep, every night. Poor sleep is one of the strongest risk factors for weight gain, so taking care of your sleep is important.

Summary : It is most important to stick to the three rules, but there are a few other things you can do to speed things up.

You can expect to lose 3-5 kilograms of weight (sometimes more) in the first week, then consistent weight loss after that.

I can personally lose 1.5 - 2 kg per week for a few weeks when I do this strictly.

If you're new to dieting, then things will probably happen quickly. The more weight you have to lose, the faster you will lose it.

For the first few days, you might feel a bit strange. Your body has been burning carbs for all these years, it can take time for it to get used to burning fat instead.

It is called the "low carb flu" and is usually over within a few days. For me it takes 3. Adding some sodium to your diet can help with this, such as dissolving a bouillon cube in a cup of hot water and drinking it.

After that, most people report feeling very good, positive and energetic. At this point you will officially have become a "fat burning beast."

Despite the decades of anti-fat hysteria, the low-carb diet also improves your health in many other ways:

Blood Sugar tends to go way down on low-carb diets..

Triglycerides tend to go down.
Small, dense LDL (the bad) Cholesterol goes down.

HDL (the good) cholesterol goes up.

Blood pressure improves significantly .
To top it all off, low-carb diets appear to be easier to follow than low-fat diets.

Summary : You can expect to lose a lot of weight, but it depends on the person how quickly it will happen. Low-carb diets also improve your health in many other ways.

You Don't Need to Starve Yourself to Lose Weight

If you have a medical condition then talk to your doctor before making changes because this plan can reduce your need for medication.

By reducing carbs and lowering insulin levels, you change the hormonal environment and make your body and brain "want" to lose weight.

This leads to drastically reduced appetite and hunger, eliminating the main reason that most people fail with conventional weight loss methods.

This is proven to make you lose about 2-3 times as much weight as a typical low-fat, calorie restricted diet.

Another great benefit for the impatient folks is that the initial drop in water weight can lead to a big difference on the scale as early as the next morning.

What foods you should eat depends on a few things, including how healthy you are, how much you exercise and how much weight you have to lose.

Foods to Avoid

You should avoid these 7 foods, in order of importance:

Sugar: Soft drinks, fruit juices, agave, candy, ice cream and many others.
Gluten Grains: Wheat, spelt, barley and rye. Includes breads and pastas.
Trans Fats: "Hydrogenated" or "partially hydrogenated" oils.
High Omega-6 Seed- and Vegetable Oils: Cottonseed-, soybean-, sunflower-, grapeseed-, corn-, safflower and canola oils.
Artificial Sweeteners: Aspartame, Saccharin, Sucralose, Cyclamates and Acesulfame Potassium. Use Stevia instead.
"Diet" and "Low-Fat" Products: Many dairy products, cereals, crackers, etc.
Highly Processed Foods: If it looks like it was made in a factory, don't eat it.

You MUST read ingredients lists, even on foods labelled as "health foods."

Low Carb Food List – Foods to Eat

You should base your diet on these real, unprocessed, low-carb foods.

Meat: Beef, lamb, pork in moderation, chicken and others. Grass-fed is best.
Fish: Salmon, trout, haddock and many others. Wild-caught fish is best.
Eggs: Omega-3 enriched or pastured eggs are best.
Vegetables: Spinach, broccoli, cauliflower, carrots and many others.
Fruits: Apples, oranges, pears, blueberries, strawberries.
Nuts and Seeds: Almonds, walnuts, sunflower seeds, etc.
High-Fat Dairy: Cheese, butter, heavy cream, yogurt.
Fats and Oils: Coconut oil, butter, lard, olive oil and cod fish liver oil.

If you need to lose weight, be careful with the cheese and nuts because they're easy to overeat on. Don't eat more than one piece of fruit per day.

Maybe Eat

If you're healthy, active and don't need to lose weight then you can afford to eat a bit more carbs.

Tubers: Potatoes, sweet potatoes and some others.
Non-gluten grains: Rice, oats, quinoa and many others.
Legumes: Lentils, black beans, pinto beans, etc. (If you can tolerate them).
You can have these in moderation if you want:

Dark Chocolate: Choose organic brands with 70% cocoa or higher.
Wine: Choose dry wines with no added sugar or carbs.
Dark chocolate is high in antioxidants and may provide health benefits if you eat it in moderation. However, be aware that both dark chocolate and alcohol will hinder your progress if you eat/drink too much.

What To Drink

Herbal Tea
Water
Sugar-free carbonated beverages, like sparkling water.
A Sample Low-Carb Menu For One Week

This is a sample menu for one week on a low carb diet plan.

It provides less than 50 grams of total carbs per day, but as I mentioned above if you are healthy and active you can go beyond that.

Monday

Breakfast: Omelet with various vegetables, fried in butter or coconut oil.
Lunch: Grass-fed yogurt with blueberries and a handful of almonds.
Dinner: Cheeseburger (no bun), served with vegetables and salsa sauce.

Tuesday

Breakfast: Bacon and eggs.
Lunch: Leftover burgers and veggies from the night before.
Dinner: Salmon with butter and vegetables.

Wednesday

Breakfast: Eggs and vegetables, fried in butter or coconut oil.
Lunch: Shrimp salad with some olive oil.
Dinner: Grilled chicken with vegetables.

Thursday

Breakfast: Omelet with various vegetables, fried in butter or coconut oil.
Lunch: Smoothie with coconut milk, berries, almonds and protein powder.
Dinner: Steak and veggies.

Friday

Breakfast: Bacon and Eggs.
Lunch: Chicken salad with some olive oil.
Dinner: Pork chops with vegetables.

Saturday

Breakfast: Omelet with various veggies.
Lunch: Grass-fed yogurt with berries, coconut flakes and a handful of walnuts.
Dinner: Meatballs with vegetables.

Sunday

Breakfast: Bacon and Eggs.
Lunch: Smoothie with coconut milk, a bit of heavy cream, chocolate-flavoured protein powder and berries.
Dinner: Grilled chicken wings with some raw spinach on the side.

If you are in Africa check below for a sample of a week's menu diet plan

Include plenty of low-carb vegetables in your diet. If your goal is to remain under 50 grams of carbs per day, then there is room for plenty of veggies and one fruit per day.

Again, if you're healthy, lean and active, you can add some tubers like potatoes and sweet potatoes, as well as some healthier grains like rice and oats.

Some Healthy, Low-Carb Snacks

There is no health reason to eat more than 3 meals per day, but if you get hungry between meals then here are some healthy, easy to prepare low-carb snacks that can fill you up:

A Piece of Fruit
Full-fat Yogurt
A Hard-Boiled Egg or Two
Baby Carrots
Leftovers From The Night Before

A Handful of Nuts
Some Cheese and Meat

Eating at Restaurants

At most restaurants, it is fairly easy to make your meals low carb-friendly.

Order a meat- or fish-based main dish.
Ask them to fry your food in real butter. though I prefer my food never fired.
Get extra vegetables instead of bread, potatoes or rice.

A Simple Low-Carb Shopping List

A good rule is to shop at the perimeter of the store, where the whole foods are likelier to be found.

Organic and grass-fed foods are best, but only if you can easily afford them. Even if you don't buy organic, your diet will still be a thousand times better than the standard western diet.

Try to choose the least processed option that still fits into your price range.

Meat (Beef, lamb, pork, chicken, bacon)
Fish (Fatty fish like salmon is best)

Eggs (Choose Omega-3 enriched or pastured eggs if you can)
Butter
Coconut Oil
Lard
Olive Oil
Cheese
Heavy Cream
Sour Cream
Yogurt (full-fat, unsweetened)
Blueberries (can be bought frozen)
Nuts
Olives
Fresh vegetables: greens, peppers, onions, etc.
Frozen vegetables: broccoli, carrots, various mixes.
Salsa Sauce
Condiments: sea salt, pepper, garlic, mustard, etc.

I recommend clearing your pantry of all unhealthy temptations if you can: chips, candy, ice cream, sodas, juices, breads, cereals and baking ingredients like wheat flour and sugar.

There is an entire world of information out there on low-carb eating. Just google "low carb recipes" or "paleo recipes" and you will find a ton of stuff.

Start losing weight with weekly meal plans based on weight loss friendly foods.

Different foods go through different metabolic pathways in the body.

They can have vastly different effects on hunger, hormones and how many calories we burn.

Here are the 20 most weight loss friendly foods on earth, that are supported by science.

1. Whole Eggs

Once feared for being high in cholesterol, whole eggs have been making a comeback.

New studies show that they don't adversely affect blood cholesterol and don't cause heart attacks.

What's more... they are among the best foods you can eat if you need to lose weight.

They're high in protein, healthy fats, and can make you feel full with a very low amount of calories.

One study of 30 overweight women showed that eating eggs for breakfast, instead of bagels, increased satiety and made them eat less for the next 36 hours.

Another 8 week study found that eggs for breakfast increased weight loss on a calorie restricted diet compared to bagels.

Eggs are also incredibly nutrient dense and can help you get all the nutrients you need on a calorie restricted diet. Almost all the nutrients are found in the yolks.

2. Leafy Greens

Leafy greens include kale, spinach, collards, swiss chards and a few others.

They have several properties that make them perfect for a weight loss diet.

They are low in both calories and carbohydrates, but loaded with fiber.

Eating leafy greens is a great way to increase the volume of your meals, without increasing the calories. Numerous studies show that meals and diets with a low energy density make people eat fewer calories overall.

Leafy greens are also incredibly nutritious and very high in all sorts of vitamins, minerals and antioxidants. This includes calcium, which has been shown to aid fat burning in some studies.

3. Salmon

Oily fish like salmon is incredibly healthy.

It is also very satisfying, keeping you full for many hours with relatively few calories.

Salmon is loaded with high quality protein, healthy fats and also contains all sorts of important nutrients.

Fish, and seafood in general, supplies a significant amount of iodine.

This nutrient is necessary for proper function of the thyroid, which is important to keep the metabolism running optimally.

Studies show that a huge number of people in the world aren't getting all the iodine they need.

Salmon is also loaded with Omega-3 fatty acids, which have been shown to help reduce inflammation, which is known to play a major role in obesity and metabolic disease.

Mackerel, trout, sardines, herring and other types of oily fish are also excellent.

4. Cruciferous Vegetables

Cruciferous vegetables include broccoli, cauliflower, cabbage and brussels sprouts.

Like other vegetables, they are high in fiber and tend to be incredibly fulfilling.

What's more... these types of veggies also tend to contain decent amounts of protein.

They're not as high in protein as animal foods or legumes, but they're high compared to most vegetables.

A combination of protein, fiber and low energy density makes cruciferous vegetables the perfect foods to include in your meals if you need to lose weight.

They are also highly nutritious, and contain cancer fighting substances.

5. Lean Beef and Chicken Breast

Meat has been unfairly demonized.

It has been blamed for all sorts of health problems, despite no good evidence to back it up.

Although processed meat is unhealthy, studies show that unprocessed red meat does NOT raise the risk of heart disease or diabetes. .

According to two big review studies, red meat has only a very weak correlation with cancer in men, and no correlation at all in women.

The truth is... meat is a weight loss friendly food, because it's high in protein.

Protein is the most fulfilling nutrient, by far, and eating a high protein diet can make you burn up to 80 to 100 more calories per day.

Studies have shown that increasing your protein intake to 25-30% of calories can cut cravings by 60%, reduce desire for late-night snacking by half, and cause weight loss of almost a pound per week... just by adding protein to the diet.

If you're on a low-carb diet, then feel free to eat fatty meats. But if you're on a moderate- to high carbohydrate diet, then choosing lean meats may be more appropriate.

6. Boiled Potatoes

White potatoes seem to have fallen out of favour for some reason.

However... they have several properties that make them a perfect food, both for weight loss and optimal health.

They contain an incredibly diverse range of nutrients, a little bit of almost everything we need.

There have even been accounts of people living on nothing but potatoes alone for extended periods of time.

They are particularly high in potassium, a nutrient that most people don't get enough of and plays an important role in blood pressure control.

On a scale called the Satiety Index, that measures how fulfilling different foods are, white, boiled potatoes scored the highest of all the foods tested..

What this means is that by eating white, boiled potatoes, you will naturally feel full and eat less of other foods instead.

If you boil the potatoes, then allow them to cool for a while, then they will form large amounts of resistant starch, a fiber-like substance that has been shown to have all sorts of health benefits... including weight loss.

Sweet potatoes, turnips and other root vegetables are also excellent.

7. Tuna

Tuna is another low-calorie, high protein food.

It is lean fish... so there isn't much fat in it.

Tuna is popular among bodybuilders and fitness models who are on a cut, because it's a great way to keep protein high, with total calories and fat low.

If you're trying to emphasize protein intake, then make sure to choose tuna canned in water, but not oil.

8. Beans and Legumes

Some beans and legumes can be beneficial for weight loss.

This includes lentils, black beans, kidney beans and some others.

These foods tend to be high in protein and fiber, which are two nutrients that have been shown to lead to satiety.

They also tend to contain some resistant starch.

The main problem is that a lot of people have problem tolerating legumes. For this reason, it is important to prepare them properly.

9. Soups

As mentioned above, meals and diets with a low energy density tend to make people eat fewer calories.

Most foods with a low energy density are those that contain lots of water, such as vegetables and fruits.

But you can also just add water to your food... by making a soup.

Some studies have shown that eating the exact same food, except made in a soup instead of as solid food, makes people feel more satiated and eat significantly fewer calories.

10. Cottage Cheese

Dairy products tend to be high in protein.

One of the best ones is cottage cheese... calorie for calorie, it is mostly just protein with very little carbohydrate and fat.

Eating plenty of cottage cheese is a great way to boost your protein intake. It is also very satiating, making you feel full with a relatively low amount of calories.

Dairy products are also high in calcium, which has been shown to aid in the fat burning process.

11. Avocados

Avocados are a unique type of fruit.

Whereas most fruit is high in carbs, avocados are loaded with healthy fats.

They are particularly high in monounsaturated oleic acid, the same type of fat found in olive oil.

Despite being mostly fat, they also contain a lot of water, so they aren't as energy dense as you may think.

Avocados are perfect as additions to salad, because studies show that the fats in them can increase the nutrient uptake from the vegetables 2.6 to 15-fold .

They also contain many important nutrients, including fiber and potassium.

12. Apple Cider Vinegar

Apple cider vinegar is incredibly popular in the natural health community.

It is popular for use in condiments, like dressings or vinaigrettes. Some people even dilute it in water and drink it.

Several studies in humans suggest that vinegar can be useful for weight loss.

Taking vinegar at the same time as a high-carb meal can increase feelings of fullness and make people eat 200-275 fewer calories for the rest of the day.

One study in obese individuals also showed that 15 or 30 mL of vinegar per day for 12 weeks caused weight loss of 2.6-3.7 pounds, or 1.2-1.7 kilograms.

Vinegar has also been shown to reduce blood sugar spikes after meals, which may lead to all sorts of beneficial effects on health in the long term.

13. Nuts

Despite being high in fat, nuts are not inherently fattening.

They're an excellent snack, containing balanced amounts of protein, fiber and healthy fats.

Studies have shown that eating nuts can improve metabolic health and even cause weight loss

Population studies have also shown that people who eat nuts tend to be healthier, and leaner, than the people who don't.

Just make sure not to go overboard, as they are still pretty high in calories. If you tend to binge and eat massive amounts of nuts, then it may be best to avoid them.

14. Some Whole Grains

Despite grains having gotten a bad rap in recent years, there are some types that are definitely healthy.

This includes some whole grains that are loaded with fiber and contain a decent amount of protein as well.

Notable examples include buckwheat, oats, brown rice and quinoa.

Buckwheat is regarded as one of the world's best food.

Oats are loaded with beta-glucans, soluble fibers that have been shown to increase satiety and improve metabolic health.

Rice, both brown and white, can also contain significant amounts of resistant starch, especially if cooked and then allowed to cool afterwards.

Keep in mind that refined grains are a disaster, and sometimes foods that have "whole grains" on the label are highly processed junk foods that are both harmful and fattening.

If you're on a very low-carb diet then you'll want to avoid grains, because they are high in carbohydrates. But there's nothing wrong with eating some of the healthier grains if you can tolerate them and are not on a low-carb diet.

15. Chili Pepper

Eating chili peppers may be useful on a weight loss diet.

They contain a substance called capsaicin, which has been shown to help reduce appetite and increase fat burning in some studies.

This substance is even sold in supplement form and is a common ingredient in many commercial weight loss supplements.

One study showed that eating 1 gram of red chilli pepper reduced appetite and increased fat burning in people who didn't regularly eat peppers.

However, there was no effect in people who were accustomed to eating spicy food, indicating that some sort of tolerance can build up.

16. Fruit

Numerous population studies have shown that people who eat the most fruit (and vegetables) tend to be healthier than people who don't.

Of course... correlation does not equal causation, so those studies don't prove anything, but fruit do have properties that make them weight loss friendly.

Even though they contain sugar, they have a low energy density and take a while to chew. Plus, the fiber helps prevent the sugar from being released too quickly into the bloodstream.

The only people who may want to avoid or minimize fruit are those who are on a very low-carb, ketogenic diet, or have some sort of intolerance to fructose.

For the rest of us, fruits can be an effective (and delicious) addition to a weight loss diet.

17. Grapefruit

One fruit that deserves to be highlighted is grapefruit, because its effects on weight control have been studied directly.

In a study of 91 obese individuals, eating half a fresh grapefruit before meals caused weight loss of 3.5 pounds (1.6 kg) over a period of 12 weeks.

The grapefruit group also had reductions in insulin resistance, a metabolic abnormality that is implicated in various chronic diseases.

So... eating half a grapefruit about a half hour before some of your daily meals may help you feel more satiated and eat fewer overall calories.

18. Chia Seeds or flax seeds

Chia seeds are among the most nutritious foods on the planet.

They do contain 12 grams of carbohydrate per ounce, which is pretty high, but 11 of those grams are fiber.

This makes chia seeds a low-carb friendly food, and one of the best sources of fiber in the world.

Because of all the fiber, chia seeds can absorb up to 11-12 times their weight in water, turning gel-like and expanding in your stomach.

Although some studies have shown that chia seeds can help reduce appetite, they have not found a statistically significant effect on weight loss.

However, given their nutrient composition, it makes sense that chia seeds could be a useful part of a weight loss diet.

19. Coconut Oil

Not all fats are created equal.

Coconut oil is high in fatty acids of a medium length, called Medium Chain Triglycerides (MCTs).

These fatty acids have been shown to boost satiety compared to other fats, as well as increase the amount of calories burned.

There are also two studies, one in women and the other in men, showing that coconut oil led to reduced amounts of belly fat.

Of course... coconut oil still contains calories, so adding it on top of what you're already eating is a bad idea.

So this is not about adding coconut oil to your diet, it is about replacing some of your other cooking fats with coconut oil.

Extra virgin olive oil is also worth mentioning here, because it is probably the healthiest fat on the planet.

20. Full-fat Yoghurt

Another excellent dairy food is yoghurt.

Yoghurt contains probiotic bacteria that can improve the function of your gut.

Having a healthy gut may potentially help protect against inflammation and leptin resistance, which is the main hormonal driver of obesity.

Just make sure to choose full-fat yoghurt... studies show that full-fat dairy, but not low-fat, is associated with a reduced risk of obesity and type 2 diabetes over time.

Low-fat yoghurt is usually loaded with sugar, so it is best to avoid that stuff like the plague.

Need to lose weight?

Start losing weight with weekly meal plans based on weight loss friendly foods.

First, soluble fiber helps regulate hormones involved in appetite control.

Some studies have found that eating soluble fiber reduces the number of hunger hormones produced by the body, including ghrelin and neuropeptide Y.

Others have shown that soluble fiber increases the production of hormones that make you feel full, such as cholecystokinin, GLP-1 and peptide YY.

Second, fiber can reduce appetite by slowing the movement of food through the gut.

When nutrients like glucose are released slowly into the gut, your body releases insulin at a slower rate. This is linked to a reduced sense of hunger.

Summary: Losing weight can help you lose belly fat. Soluble fiber can help you lose weight by curbing your appetite, which reduces calorie intake.
Sources of Soluble Fiber

Soluble fiber is easy to add to your diet and found in a variety of plant-based foods.

Foods that are high in soluble fiber include flaxseeds, sweet potatoes, fruits like apricots and oranges, Brussels sprouts, legumes and grains like oatmeal.

However, although soluble fiber may help you lose belly fat, it's not a great idea to eat lots of soluble fiber right away.

This can cause side effects, such as stomach cramps, diarrhea and bloating. It's best to increase your intake slowly, over time, to help improve your body's tolerance.

As far as recommended daily intake goes, the US Department of Agriculture recommends that men aim to consume 30–38 grams of fiber per day, while women should aim for 21–25 grams per day.

Summary: Great sources of soluble fiber include flaxseeds, legumes, grains, fruits and vegetables. Aim to increase your intake slowly over time.

Ketogenic diet

Ketogenic diet (keto) is a low-carb, high-fat diet. It lowers blood sugar and insulin levels, and shifts the body's metabolism away from carbs and towards fat and ketones.

A ketogenic diet can help you lose much more weight than a low-fat diet. This often happens without hunger.

Different Types of Ketogenic Diets

There are several versions of the ketogenic diet, including:

Standard ketogenic diet (SKD): This is a very low-carb, moderate-protein and high-fat diet. It typically contains 75% fat, 20% protein and only 5% carbs.
Cyclical ketogenic diet (CKD): This diet involves periods of higher-carb refeeds, such as 5 ketogenic days followed by 2 high-carb days.
Targeted ketogenic diet (TKD): This diet allows you to add carbs around workouts.
High-protein ketogenic diet: This is similar to a standard ketogenic diet, but includes more protein. The ratio is often 60% fat, 35% protein and 5% carbs.
However, only the standard and high-protein ketogenic diets have been studied extensively. Cyclical or targeted ketogenic diets are more advanced methods, and primarily used by bodybuilders or athletes.

The information in this writing mostly applies to the standard ketogenic diet (SKD), although many of the same principles also apply to the other versions.

There are several versions of the ketogenic diet. The standard ketogenic diet (SKD) is the most researched.

Summary :The ketogenic diet can boost insulin sensitivity and cause fat loss, leading to drastic improvement for type 2 diabetes and prediabetes.

Other Health Benefits of the Ketogenic Diet

The ketogenic diet actually originated as a tool for treating neurological diseases, such as epilepsy.

Studies have now shown that the diet can have benefits for a wide variety of different health conditions:

Heart disease: The ketogenic diet can improve risk factors like body fat, HDL levels, blood pressure and blood sugar.

Cancer: The diet is currently being used to treat several types of cancer and slow tumor growth.

Alzheimer's disease: The diet may reduce symptoms of Alzheimer's and slow down the disease's progression.

Epilepsy: Research has shown that the ketogenic diet can cause massive reductions in seizures in epileptic children.

Parkinson's disease: One study found that the diet helped improve symptoms of Parkinson's disease.

Polycystic ovary syndrome: The ketogenic diet can help reduce insulin levels, which may play a key role in polycystic ovary syndrome.

Brain injuries: One animal study found that the diet can reduce concussions and aid recovery after brain injury.

Acne: Lower insulin levels and eating less sugar or processed foods may help improve acne.

However, keep in mind that research into many of these areas is far from conclusive.

Summary : A ketogenic diet may provide many health benefits, especially with metabolic, neurological or insulin-related diseases.

Foods to Avoid

In short, any food that is high in carbs should be limited.

Here is a list of foods that need to be reduced or eliminated on a ketogenic diet:

Sugary foods: Soda, fruit juice, smoothies, cake, ice cream, candy, etc.
Grains or starches: Wheat-based products, rice, pasta, cereal, etc.

Fruit: All fruit, except small portions of berries like strawberries.

Beans or legumes: Peas, kidney beans, lentils, chickpeas, etc.

Root vegetables and tubers: Potatoes, sweet potatoes, carrots, parsnips, etc.

Low-fat or diet products: These are highly processed and often high in carbs.

Some condiments or sauces: These often contain sugar and unhealthy fat.

Unhealthy fat: Limit your intake of processed vegetable oils, mayonnaise, etc.

Alcohol: Due to its carb content, many alcoholic beverages can throw you out of ketosis.

Sugar-free diet foods: These are often high in sugar alcohols, which can affect ketone levels in some cases. These foods also tend to be highly processed.

Summary : Avoid carb-based foods like grains, sugars, legumes, rice, potatoes, candy, juice and even most fruits.

Foods to Eat

You should base the majority of your meals around these foods:

Meat: Red meat, steak, ham, sausage, bacon, chicken and turkey.

Fatty fish: Such as salmon, trout, tuna and mackerel.

Eggs: Look for pastured or omega-3 whole eggs.

Butter and cream: Look for grass-fed when possible.

Cheese: Unprocessed cheese (cheddar, goat, cream, blue or mozzarella).
Nuts and seeds: Almonds, walnuts, flaxseeds, pumpkin seeds, chia seeds, etc.

Healthy oils: Primarily extra virgin olive oil, coconut oil and avocado oil.

Avocados: Whole avocados or freshly made guacamole.

Low-carb veggies: Most green veggies, tomatoes, onions, peppers, etc.

Condiments: You can use salt, pepper and various healthy herbs and spices.
It is best to base your diet mostly on whole, single ingredient foods.

Summary : Base the majority of your diet on foods such as meat, fish, eggs, butter, nuts, healthy oils, avocados and plenty of low-carb veggies.

A Sample Ketogenic Meal Plan For 1 Week

PS: If you are an African and you cannot do without 'swallow' then find a substitute for those starchy stuffs we swallow (that is, if you are on a weight loss journey).

There are also tons of fruits , vegetables, spices and roots that are edible and can as well enhance weight loss. Make google your friend :)

In whichever country or continent you are, always go for seasonal food products

To help get you started, here is a sample ketogenic diet meal plan for one week:

Monday

Breakfast: Bacon, eggs and tomatoes.
Lunch: Chicken salad with olive oil and feta cheese.
Dinner: Salmon with asparagus cooked in butter.

Tuesday

Breakfast: Egg, tomato, basil and goat cheese omelet.
Lunch: Almond milk, peanut butter, cocoa powder and stevia milkshake.
Dinner: Meatballs, cheddar cheese and vegetables.

Wednesday

Breakfast: A ketogenic milkshake
Lunch: Shrimp salad with olive oil and avocado.
Dinner: Pork chops with Parmesan cheese, broccoli and salad.

Thursday

Breakfast: Omelet with avocado, salsa, peppers, onion and spices.
Lunch: A handful of nuts and celery sticks with guacamole and salsa.
Dinner: Chicken stuffed with pesto and cream cheese, along with vegetables.

Friday

Breakfast: Sugar-free yogurt with peanut butter, cocoa powder and stevia.
Lunch: Beef stir-fry cooked in coconut oil with vegetables.
Dinner: Burger with bacon, egg and cheese.

Saturday

Breakfast: Ham and cheese omelet with vegetables.
Lunch: Ham and cheese slices with nuts.
Dinner: White fish, egg and spinach cooked in coconut oil.

Sunday

Breakfast: Fried eggs with bacon and mushrooms.
Lunch: Burger with salsa, cheese and guacamole.
Dinner: Steak and eggs with a side salad.

Always try to rotate the vegetables and meat over the long term, as each type provides different nutrients and health benefits.

Be creative. Create your own menu with with equivalent food products that are seasonal and most available in your area.

It is better that you avoid frying of any sort.

Summary : You can eat a wide variety of tasty and nutritious meals on a ketogenic diet.

Healthy Ketogenic Snacks

In case you get hungry between meals, here are some healthy, keto-approved snacks:

Fatty meat or fish.
Cheese.
A handful of nuts or seeds.
Cheese with olives.
1–2 hard-boiled eggs.
90% dark chocolate.
A low-carb milk shake with almond milk, cocoa powder and nut butter.
Full-fat yogurt mixed with nut butter and cocoa powder.
Strawberries and cream.
Celery with salsa and guacamole.
Smaller portions of leftover meals.
Bottom Line: Great snacks for a keto diet include pieces of meat, cheese, olives, boiled eggs, nuts and dark chocolate.

Side Effects and How to Minimize Them

Although the ketogenic diet is safe for healthy people, there may be some initial side effects while your body adapts.

This is often referred to as "keto flu" – and is usually over within a few days.

Eating more fat at this time instead of carbs or protein will help, if we really want to lose weight.

Low Carb plans such as Atkins can be very effective for some people including me, many people who start a low carb diet experience get what's called the "ketosis flu" or the "induction flu" in the first few days while the body is adapting to burning ketones instead of glucose.

The basic symptoms are:
– Headaches
– Nausea
– Upset stomach
– Lack of mental clarity (brain fog)
– Sleepiness
– Fatigue

It's called the "ketosis flu" for a reason: you feel sick. I've gone through it and it wasn't a pleasant experience. Fortunately it only lasted 2 days but then suddenly I woke up feeling much better, less hungry and my energy level was really high and consistent throughout the day!

The first time I thought to myself: "What the heck am I doing? I feel like I'm going to die!" but I persevered and when it was over I didn't regret a thing because what I had gained mentally and physically was 100% worth it.

For those of you that are going through the ketosis flu, don't give up! I know you feel like it's never going to get better but stick with it and you´ll be so happy you did!

 I'm telling you, waking up refreshed for the first time in years, not getting the afternoon "blah" feeling and stuffing my face with carbs to try to boost my energy is the best side effect of the low carb diet I've experienced. Okay, losing weight while eating good food, feeling full and satisfied is great too.

First you have to understand why your body is reacting this way. Your body's been burning glucose for energy so it's basically full of enzymes that are waiting to deal with the carbs you eat, but now the body needs to make new enzymes that burn fat for fuel instead of carbs, and the transition period causes the flu-like symptoms.

There are some things you can do to lessen the symptoms of the ketosis flu and to make it go away sooner (to force the body to transition sooner) Ok, let's get to the good part – what to do:

First of all – you're probably dehydrated. Drink PLENTY of water while you're on a low carb diet, and then drink some more.

Watch your electrolytes. When the body is getting rid of excess insulin from your former carb-crazy diet you´ll lose lots of fluids that have been retained in your body.

This causes the rapid weight loss most people see in their first few days of ketosis, it's mostly water, sorry. When you lose all the retained water you also lose electrolytes like sodium, magnesium and potassium.

When you're lacking them you´ll feel like crap so when you're feeling really ill on the ketosis flu try things like chicken/beef broth and look for foods rich in these minerals. Take a multi-vitamin and a multi-mineral.

Ok, here is where people throw the red flag – Eat more fat – Yeah, I said MORE fat. Have some butter, just not on a roll, eat some bacon and eggs for breakfast, just skip the potatoes and toast. This will force your body to hurry up the transition. You´ll think this is crazy and think you´ll never get lose weight eating this way, but you will.

Don't eat too much protein – The body can transform protein into glucose so if you eat too much of it in the first days it will slow down the transition.

Go for fatty meat and cheese if you can, add fat to protein shakes etc.

Drink water, replenish electrolytes (sodium, magnesium, potassium) with food and supplements, drink broth, eat fat and not too much protein.

Keto flu includes poor energy and mental function, increased hunger, sleep issues, nausea, digestive discomfort and decreased exercise performance.

In order to minimize this, you can try a regular low-carb diet for the first few weeks. This may teach your body to burn more fat before you completely eliminate carbs.

A ketogenic diet can also change the water and mineral balance of your body, so adding extra salt to your meals or taking mineral supplements can help.

For minerals, try taking 3,000–4,000 mg of sodium, 1,000 mg of potassium and 300 mg of magnesium per day to minimize side effects.

At least in the beginning, it is important to eat until fullness and to avoid restricting calories too much. Usually a ketogenic diet causes weight loss without intentional calorie restriction.

Summary : Many of the side effects of starting a ketogenic diet can be limited. Easing into the diet and taking mineral supplements can help.

Frequently Asked Questions

Here are answers to some of the most common questions about the ketogenic diet.

1. Can I ever eat carbs again?

Yes. However, it is important to eliminate them initially. After the first 2–3 months, you can eat carbs on special occasions — just return to the diet immediately after.

2. Will I lose muscle?

There is a risk of losing some muscle on any diet. However, the high protein intake and high ketone levels may help minimize muscle loss, especially if you lift weights.

3. Can you build muscle on a ketogenic diet?

Yes, but it may not work as well as on a moderate-carb diet. More details: Low-Carb/Ketogenic Diets and Exercise Performance.

4. Do I need to refeed or carb load?

No. However, a few higher-calorie days may be beneficial every now and then.

5. How much protein can I eat?

Protein should be moderate, as a very high intake can spike insulin levels and lower ketones. Around 35% of total calorie intake is probably the upper limit.

6. What if I am constantly tired, weak or fatigued?

You may not be in full ketosis or be utilizing fats and ketones efficiently. To counter this, lower your carb intake and re-visit the points above.

7. My urine smells fruity? Why is this?

Don't be alarmed. This is simply due to the excretion of byproducts created during ketosis.

8. My breath smells. What can I do?

This is a common side effect. Try drinking naturally flavored water or chewing sugar-free gum.

9. I heard ketosis was extremely dangerous. Is this true?

People often confuse ketosis with ketoacidosis. The former is natural, while the latter only occurs in uncontrolled diabetes.

Ketoacidosis is dangerous, but the ketosis on a ketogenic diet is perfectly normal and healthy.

10. I have digestion issues and diarrhea. What can I do?

This common side effect usually passes after 3–4 weeks. If it persists, try eating more high-fiber veggies. Magnesium supplements can also help with constipation.

A Ketogenic Diet is Great, But Not For Everyone

A ketogenic diet can be great for people who are overweight, diabetic or looking to improve their metabolic health.

It may be less suitable for elite athletes or those wishing to add large amounts of muscle or weight.

And, as with any diet, it will only work if you are consistent and stick with it in the long-term.

That being said, few things are as well proven in nutrition as the powerful health and weight loss benefits of a ketogenic diet.

The content in this book is intended for informational and educational purposes only. Consult a doctor for medical advice, treatment or diagnosis.

Surprise! Surprise! Here is my gift gift! Click on the link below:

https://youtu.be/UUtM59Y4WXE - Enjoy this simple tips too on how to shed some fat. Like share and subscribe to my YouTube Channel.
 Thank You

Nkiru Ojimadu
A Multi Award Winning Personality
Life Transformational Coach,
Best Selling Author,
International Speaker.
Co-Founder Relationships 101.
TV Host.

Follow me on social media

Facebook: nkiru ojimadu (niki)
Instagram: nikioj
Twitter: nikioj
YouTube: nkiru ojimadu

To get my books just type "Nkiru Ojimadu" on Amazon or Okadabooks

www.ingramcontent.com/pod-product-compliance
Lightning Source LLC
Chambersburg PA
CBHW072016290526
45787CB00013B/942